Clean Eating Slow Cooking
19 Days of Clean Eating Slow Cooker Recipes

By S.J. Blackman

Copyright: Published in the United States by S.J. Blackman / © S.J. Blackman

Published 09/08/2015

All rights reserved. No part of this publication may be reproduced, stored in retrieval system, copied in any form or by any means, electronic, mechanical, photocopying, recording or otherwise transmitted without written permission from the publisher. Please do not participate in or encourage piracy of this material in any way. You must not circulate this book in any format. S.J. Blackman does not control or direct users' actions and is not responsible for the information or content shared, harm and/or actions of the book readers.

In accordance with the U.S. Copyright Act of 1976, the scanning, uploading and electronic sharing of any part of this book without the permission of the publisher constitute unlawful piracy and theft of the author's intellectual property. If you would like to use material from the book (other than just simply for reviewing the book), prior permission must be obtained by contacting the author.

Thank you for your support of the author's rights.

Many individuals have become confused into believing that clean eating is a diet. This way of eating is not something you do for a couple of months and then return back to processed or artificial foods. Developing a clean eating regimen is a lifestyle change.

Clean eating is not about depriving yourself but making smarter food choices. There are tons of great clean eating recipes out there, however, we have compiled a great collection of clean eating slow cooker recipes to suit your appetite and help you to save time and energy in the kitchen.

Additional Reads and Recommendations

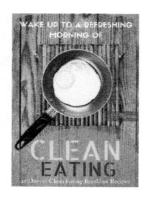

Wake Up to a Refreshing Morning of Clean Eating: 25 Days of Clean Eating Breakfast Recipes

Clean Eating: Amazingly Delicious Recipes To Jump Start Your Weight Loss, Increase Energy and Feel Great! (Clean Food Diet Book 1)

Clean Eating: Clean Eating Diet: The 7-Day Plan for Weight Loss & Delicious Recipes for Clean Eating Diet (Clean Eating, Weight Loss, Healthy Diet, Healthy ... Paleo Diet, Lose Weight Fast, Flat Belly)

Table of Contents

1. What Does It Mean To Go Clean?

2. Maintain Good Clean Eating Habits

3. Southwestern Black Bean Chicken

4. Orange Peel Cornish Hens

5. Pork Roast and Vegetable Stew

6. Corn Tortilla Chicken Stew

7. Kale and Pork Loin Chops

8. Turkey Meatballs and Kale

9. Asian Chicken Drumsticks

10. Ginger Sesame Seed Chicken

11. Spicy Sriracha Beef & Bell Pepper

12. Lentils and Brown Rice

13. Cajun Chicken Stew

14. Chunky Pineapple Chicken Curry

15. Honey Pecan Chicken

16. Slow Cooker Red Pepper Chili

17. Sweet & Spicy Chicken Tacos

18. Salsa Barbeque Chicken Tacos

19. Chicken and Dumplings

20. Spicy Italian Chicken

21. Pulled Pork Pepper & Slaw Tacos

22. Additional Reads and Recommendations

What Does It Mean To Go Clean?

To put it in simple terms, it means to consume foods as close to their natural state as possible. More individuals are becoming aware of added preservative and chemicals negatively affect their body and health over time. These individuals are seeking ways to eliminate those chemicals from their food intake diets and body. Doing this will essentially bringing their body to a better balance and healthier state.

The less ingredients in food, the closer it will be to its natural state, which makes it higher in quality. The more ingredients a food has, the more processed the food becomes along with more added preservatives and chemicals it contains.

Eating clean can be described as consuming whole, natural foods such as fruits, vegetables, lean proteins, and complex carbohydrates. By accepting a clean eating lifestyle is essential that you refrain from any junk food. Junk food contains man-made sugar, bad fats (hydrogenated, trans-fat), preservatives, and white bread. These unhealthy foods are filled

with empty calories and have zero nutritional value.

Maintain Good Clean Eating Habits

Here we have developed a list of good clean eating habits to help keep you on track and develop healthy eating choices.

- It is essential that you eliminate refined sugar from your diet.

- Be sure to read labels and select foods with fewer ingredients (3-6 ingredients).

- Develop a daily schedule to cook and prepare healthy meals to avoid impulsive unhealthy food choices.

- Stay hydrated by consuming at least 8 glasses of water a day.

- Eliminate or limit your alcoholic beverage intake.

- Develop a plan or schedule to wake up earlier enough to eat breakfast every day.

- Include plenty of fruits and vegetables into every meal.

- Exchange white carbohydrates for brown, whole grains or brown rice.

- Develop and maintain a 7 to 8 hour sleeping schedule.

- Consume protein such as chicken, fish, beef and turkey. It is an important because it causes positive release of the hormone glucagon (raises blood sugar) which counteracts the hormone insulin (lowers your blood sugar). This results in a stable blood sugar because the two hormones essentially balance each other.

- Consume foods with fiber: Fiber slows down the rate of digestion which assists with maximum blood sugar stabilization. Consume 25-35 grams of fiber per day.

- Consume good unsaturated fats. Not all fat is bad, consuming saturated fat can cause health complications. One benefit of consuming unsaturated fat is that it slows down digestion; which causes your body to release stored fat.

- Maintain good portion control. Practice healthy eating by properly balancing your meals. Every meal should contain 45-60% carbohydrates; 10-35% proteins; and 20-35% fats. Your body needs all of these essential nutrients, along with vitamins, minerals and water, in order to function properly.

Carbohydrates provide your body with the glucose it needs to feed your brain and to fuel your cells with energy; proteins are used to build and repair your body tissues; while lipids from fats provide the essential fatty acids that your body needs for your cell membranes, the production of hormones, and healthy skin. These are essential nutrients and you need them in every meal in the right proportions. If you are able to maintain these eating habits, you will be well on your way to having your body functioning at its best potential.

The key to maintaining a healthy lifestyle is to adopt some good clean eating habits. Be sure to drink more water, discard processed foods, balance your meals properly and maintain the right portion sizes. Changing the way you eat is not easy. It will take some good time and effort. It is important to make the decision to change and try your best to remain on track. Develop gradual changes by beginning with one meal at a time as opposed to doing it all at once and you will be on your way to a healthier eating lifestyle.

3. Southwestern Black Bean Chicken

Yield: 10 Servings

Ingredients:

4 raw, boneless, skinless chicken breasts (about 8 oz. each)

1 (15 ounce) can pinto beans, rinsed and drained

1 (15 ounce) can black beans, rinsed and drained

1 (28 ounce) can diced tomatoes in juice, low sodium is best

1 pound frozen and thawed organic corn

1 (12 ounce) jar of your favorite salsa, no sugar added

Directions:

- Add the chicken breasts in the slow cooker.

- Add in the tomatoes and salsa over, layer on the beans and corn.

- Cook on low for 5-7 hours, or until the chicken easily tears apart.

4. Orange Peel Cornish Hens

Yield: 2 Servings

Ingredients:

2 cornish game hens

1 medium orange

1 tsp. garlic powder

1 tsp. onion powder

1/2 tsp. ground cinnamon

1/2 tsp. ground cumin

1/8 tsp. ground cloves

Directions:

- Add the hens in the slow cooker.
- Slice the orange in half, then cut off one slice and place aside.
- Squeeze out and reserve the juice.
- In a mixing bowl, mix the spices.
- Add in 1 tbsp. of orange juice and mix to create a paste.
- Apply herbs over the game hens.
- Slice the orange slice in half, place on top of your game hens.

- Add in 2 tbsp. of orange juice to the bottom of the slow cooker.
- Cover and cook on low for 2-3 hours.

5. Pork Roast and Vegetable Stew

Yield: 6-8 Servings

Ingredients:

3 lb. bone-in pork shoulder

1 lb. baby carrots

7 oz. pearl onions

8 oz. package brown mushrooms, halved or quartered

6 oz. can tomato paste, no sugar added

2 tbsp. garlic powder

1 tbsp. dried thyme

1 tbsp. dried sage

1/4 cup balsamic vinegar

1 cup seasoned chicken broth

Directions:

- Add the roast in the slow cooker.
- Add the carrots, onions and mushrooms around the roast.
- Combine the leftover ingredients in a bowl to make the sauce, apply it over the roast and   veggies.
- Cook at low for 10 hours.
- Remove the roast and stir the tomato paste into the remaining sauce.

- Apply the sauce over everything when serving.

6. Corn Tortilla Chicken Stew

Yield: 7 Servings

Ingredients:

1 1/2 lb. raw chicken breasts

1 (12 oz.) salsa

1 pound frozen corn, thawed

1 pound frozen, mixed bell peppers

3 organic, corn tortillas, ripped or shredded by hand

Olives and yogurt for garnish (optional)

Directions:

- Add the chicken in the slow cooker.
- Apply everything else over it.
- Cook on low for 8-10 hours.
- When finished, use a wooden spoon to stir and break apart the chicken.
- Serve garnished with black olives or a bit of plain yogurt.

7. Kale and Pork Loin Chops

Yield: 9 Servings

Ingredients:

2 1/2 pounds pork loin chops

7 cups chopped, raw kale

1 (28 ounce) can diced tomatoes, no sugar added

2 tbsps. Garlic powder

1 tbsp. onion powder

1 tbsp. balsamic vinegar

Directions:

- Add all the ingredients in to the slow cooker.
- Place the pork chops on the bottom then the tomatoes on the top.
- Prepare on low for 8-10 hours.

8. Turkey Meatballs and Kale

Yield: 8 Servings

Ingredients:

¼ cup milk

2 slices bread

1 pound lean ground turkey

1 medium shallot, finely chopped

2 cloves garlic, finely chopped

½ tsp. freshly grated nutmeg

1 tsp. oregano

¼ tsp. red pepper flakes

Kosher salt and freshly ground pepper

½ cup Parmigiano-Reggiano, grated, plus more for garnish

2 tbsps. Italian parsley, chopped

1 egg, beaten

1 tbsp. olive oil

8 cups chicken or vegetable broth

1 15-ounce can white Northern beans or other small white bean, drained and rinsed

2 carrots, sliced

½ yellow onion, chopped

4 cups kale

Directions:

- Add milk in a bowl, tear the bread into chunks then add to the milk.
- Place in the turkey, shallot, garlic, nutmeg, oregano, red pepper flakes, salt and pepper, cheese, parsley and egg and mix well until the mixture is combined.
- Use a small scoop to form ½ inch balls.
- Warm the olive oil in a skillet over medium high heat.
- Slightly sear the meatballs for 1-2 minutes on both sides.
- Take away from the pan, place aside.
- Add the broth, beans, carrots, onion and kale to the slow cooker.
- Place the meatballs onto the kale, cover and cook on low for 4 hours.
- Garnish the soup with grated parmesan cheese, red pepper flakes and fresh parsley leaves.

9. Asian Chicken Drumsticks

Yield: 6-8 Servings

Ingredients:

6 tbsp. soy sauce

1/4 cup honey

1/4 cup water

4 + 1/2 tbsp. cornstarch

1 large garlic clove, crushed

2 tsp fresh ginger, grated

3 lbs. or 12 chicken drumsticks, skinless (or thighs)

3 tbsp. green onions, chopped

1 tbsp. sesame seeds

Directions:

- In the slow cooker, combine soy sauce, honey, water, cornstarch, garlic and ginger.
- Heat a non-stick skillet to low medium heat then place in chicken.
- Prepare for 3 - 4 minutes on both sides, turning once.
- Add the chicken to a slow cooker, coat the chicken in mixture.
- Cook on low setting for 6 - 8 hours or high for 3 hours.

- Once finished use tongs or a spatula to gently move the drumsticks around to coat in the sauce. Serve up with brown rice, garnished with sesame seeds and green onions.

10. Ginger Sesame Seed Chicken

Yield: 8-10 Servings

Ingredients:

4 Chicken Breasts, sliced into bite size pieces
1/2 cup Honey
3 Tbsp. Reduced Sodium Soy Sauce
1 Inch Fresh Ginger Root, Grated
2 Tbsp. Lime Juice
2 Tsp. Sesame Oil
1 Tsp. Rice Wine Vinegar
4 Garlic Cloves, Smashed
1 Medium Yellow Onion, Diced
Salt & Pepper to Taste
1 Tbsp. Cornstarch
1 Tbsp. Water

Optional Toppings:
Sesame Seeds, Green Onions, Sriracha.

Directions:

- Lightly spray the inside of your slow cooker.
- Add all the ingredients into a crock pot, except the cornstarch and water, stir.
- Prepare on low for at least 6-8 hours or high for 4-6 hours.
- Approximately 30 minutes before to serving, mix the corn starch and water.
- Add into the crock pot, stir, and allow to cook for approximately 30 minutes.
- When finishes remove the lid and stir.
- Serve over rice, noodles, or vegetables.

11. Spicy Sriracha Beef & Bell Pepper

Yield: 6-8 Servings

Ingredients:

2 lbs. beef chuck, thinly sliced

2 cups chopped to 1 inch squares bell pepper

½ medium onion, peeled, cut in half, sliced

1 cup broth or 1 cup water + 3 bouillon cubes

2 tsp freeze dried garlic

⅓ cup chopped parsley

2 tsp salt

1 tsp black pepper

½ cup water

2 tbsp. corn starch

Optional:

1 tbsp. Sriracha

Directions:

- Add the meat to the slow cooker.
- Add atop the sliced onion and cut up bell pepper.

- Sprinkle with salt, pepper and garlic.
- Mix the broth with Sriracha, or water, bouillon cubes and Sriracha.
- Apply over the peppers and beef.
- Cook at high heat for 3.5-4 hours.
- Combine ½ cup water and 2 tbsps. corn starch.
- Add in 1 cup of liquid from the meat & pepper mixture and cook on medium heat till boiling.
- Cook 2 minutes past boil to remove the cornstarch flavor.
- Place the mixture back into the meat and bell peppers.
- Add over chopped parsley, stir and serve.
- Serve over rice.

12. Lentils and Brown Rice

Yield: 8 Servings

Ingredients:

1 cup uncooked brown long grain rice

1 cup dried lentils

1 medium onion, diced

1 can (14.5 ounces) low sodium diced tomatoes

5 ounces fresh spinach, chopped or frozen, but thaw and drain first

5 cups low sodium vegetable broth

2 cloves garlic, minced

2 tsp dried oregano

1 tsp dried basil

1 tsp sea salt or to taste

1/2 tsp fresh ground black pepper or to taste

1 package (8 ounces) nondairy cheese (optional)

Directions:

- Add rice and lentils in a bowl then cover with water and for least 6 hours.
- Drain, add in the slow cooker with the ingredients except the cheese.
- Cover and cook on high 5-6 hours or low 8 hours.
- Add the cheese individually to each serving.

13. Cajun Chicken Stew

Yield: 8 Servings

Ingredients:

2 tbsps. olive oil

2 cups onion, chopped

2 cups celery, chopped

2 cups green bell pepper, chopped

6 cloves garlic, chopped

1 6-ounce can organic tomato paste

2 15-ounce cans organic chopped tomatoes

1 cup low sodium chicken broth

2 tsps. Cajun seasoning

1/4 tsp. black pepper

2 bay leaves

1 tsp. dried thyme

3 pounds skinless, boneless chicken thighs

Fresh chopped parsley and chopped scallions, for serving

Hot sauce, if desired

Directions:

- In a heated and oiled skillet add onion, celery, bell pepper, and garlic.

- Sauté on medium heat for 5-7 minutes, till fragrant.
- Add tomato paste and mix into vegetables; prepare for 2 minutes.
- Add the vegetables into slow cooker.
- Place in the chopped tomatoes, chicken broth, Cajun seasoning, pepper, bay leaves and thyme.
- Stir to mix well.
- Add chicken thighs in sauce.
- Cook on low for 4 hours.
- Serve warm.

14. Chunky Pineapple Chicken Curry

Yield: 6 Servings

Ingredients:

1 (20 oz.) can pineapple chunks in juice, drained, reserving 2 tbsps.

7 tbsp. red curry paste

3 tbsp. fish sauce

2 tbsp. fresh lime juice

2 tbsp. fresh grated ginger

1 tbsp. brown sugar

1 small white onion, halved and sliced

3 lbs. chicken breast, cut into 1-inch chunks

1/2 c. coconut milk (lite)

2 bell peppers, seeded and cut into chunks

Rice, chopped peanuts, and cilantro

Directions:

- Mix 2 tbsps. of pineapple juice, curry paste, fish sauce, lime juice, ginger, and sugar then place aside
- Add the onion across the bottom of the slow cooker.
- Position the chicken in slow cooker over onion.

- Apply the sauce over chicken.
- Prepare on low for 6-7 hours.
- Place in the coconut milk, pineapple chunks, and bell pepper sat the last 30 minutes of cooking.
- Serve over rice, garnish with chopped peanuts and cilantro, if desired.

15. Honey Pecan Chicken

Yield: 4 Servings

Ingredients:

4 chicken breasts

1 tsp. sea salt

Freshly ground black pepper

2/3 cups honey

1 cup chopped pecans

3 cloves garlic (minced)

1 tbsp. Herbs de Provence (or Italian Seasoning)

A dash of ground cinnamon

A handful of fresh Italian flat leaf parsley (chopped)

Directions:

- Apply to the chicken salt & pepper, add in slow cooker.
- In a bowl, add garlic, herbs de Provence, and cinnamon to the honey.
- Stir well and apply over the chicken.
- Sprinkle in the pecans, and prepare on low for 3-4 hours.
- Once finishes, remove chicken from crock pot and cover with aluminum foil.
- Allow to set for 5-10 minutes.

- Shred chicken or serve whole with the sauce drizzled on top with a handful of fresh parsley.
- Serve up with vegetables.

16. Slow Cooker Red Pepper Chili

Yield: 3-4 Servings

Ingredients:

2 large Red peppers, chopped

1 large Vidalia onion, chopped

3 cloves of garlic, grated or minced

1 ½ pounds of lean ground turkey

1 28 ounce can of crushed tomatoes

1 15 oz. can corn kernels, no salt added, drained

1 15 oz. can black beans, low sodium, drained

2 tsp-2 tbsp. chili powder (depending on desired spice)

1 tbsp. cumin

1 tbsp. smoked paprika

1 tbsp. onion powder

½ tbsp. salt

1 cup chicken stock

¼ cup apple cider vinegar

Toppings:

Cilantro

Tomatoes

Avocado

Directions:

- Place all of the chili ingredients in the slow cooker.
- Stir until nicely combined.
- Set the slow cooker to high for 4 hours.
- Serve warm with chopped tomatoes, cilantro and avocado.

17. Sweet & Spicy Chicken Tacos

Yield: 6-8 Servings

Ingredients:

Sweet & Spicy Chicken:

2 lbs. (4-5 count) Chicken Breasts, trimmed of fat

1 cup very warm water

¼ cup white vinegar

2 tbsp. lemon juice

2 tbsp. Worcestershire sauce

4 tbsp. melted butter

⅓ cup ketchup

⅓ cup brown sugar, lightly packed

2 tsp dry mustard

2 tsp salt

2 tsp chili powder

Toppings/ Taco accessories:

Small flour tortillas (10-12)

Lettuce, chopped

Tomatoes, diced

Cheddar cheese, shredded

Guacamole

Cilantro

Sour Cream

Hot sauce (Tabasco)

Try Fluffy Three Pepper Sausage Corn Cakes

Directions:

Prepare Chicken Tacos:

- Mix together 1 cup water, ⅓ cup ketchup, ¼ cup vinegar, 2 tbsp. lemon juice, 2 tbsp. Worcestershire sauce, 4 tbsp. melted butter, ⅓ cup brown sugar, 2 tsp dry mustard, 2 tsp salt, 2 tsp chili powder.
- Place the chicken in the slow cooker and add the marinade over the top.
- Coat in the sauce.
- Set to high for 4 hours or low for 6 hours, keep warm until ready to serve.
- Pull chicken with two forks and set in the slow cooker juices until ready to serve.

- To assemble the tacos dice, grate and chop all of your fixings.
- Warm up your tortillas between two lightly damp paper towels and microwaving for 30 seconds.
- Add the chicken then layer the rest of the toppings adding the hot sauce if preferred.

18. Salsa Barbeque Chicken Tacos

Yield: 8 Servings

Ingredients:

6 chicken breast halves (about 1.5 lbs.)

16 oz. jar salsa

6 oz. can tomato paste

2 tsp ground (dry) mustard

1/4 cup molasses

2 tbsp. Worcestershire sauce

3 tbsp. apple cider vinegar

3 tbsp. honey

Directions:

- Add all the ingredients into the slow cooker and stir.
- Prepare on high for 4 hours or on low for 6-8 hours.
- When cooled remove the chicken and shred it using two forks.
- Add the shredded chicken back into the sauce, cook for an additional 30 minutes with the lid off to thicken the sauce.
- Serve warm.

19. Chicken and Dumplings

Yield: 6-8 Servings

Stew Ingredients:

6 cups low-sodium chicken broth (no sugar/dextrose added)

1 tbsp. marjoram

1 tbsp. garlic powder

4 boneless, skinless chicken breasts sliced into small chunks

2 tbsps. olive oil

1 large onion – peeled and diced

4 large carrots, peeled and sliced

4 stalks celery, cleaned and sliced

Dumpling Ingredients:

2 cups whole wheat pastry flour

1 tbsp. baking soda

1/2 tsp. salt

3 tbsps. olive oil

1 cup milk (or unsweetened almond milk.)

Directions:

Prepare the Stew:

- Pour the broth into the slow cooker.
- Place in the marjoram and garlic powder and switch the slow cooker to high.
- In a pan, mix olive oil, onion, carrots and celery.
- Sauté till the onions are translucent.
- Add the vegetables and cut up chicken to the crock pot.

Prepare the Dumplings:

- In a bowl, mix flour, baking soda and salt and blend well.
- Pour in the oil and milk, combine with a wooden spoon.
- Scoop then round off the dumplings and scrap into your pot.
- Cook on high for approximately 3-1/2 hours.
- When finished break up the dumplings with a wooden spoon and stir them into the stew to finish cooking.

20. Spicy Italian Chicken

Yield: 10 Servings

Ingredients:

4 lbs. boneless, skinless chicken breasts

5 medium tomatoes, chopped

1 onion, chopped

3 tbsp. garlic, minced

2 tbsp. tomato paste

2 tbsp. olive oil

1 tbsp. honey

2 tbsp. Italian Seasoning

1/4 - 1 tsp. red pepper flakes

1 tsp. sea salt

1 tsp. black pepper

Directions:

- Combine all of the ingredients (except the chicken) and mix for approximately 30 seconds until all the ingredients are mixed well.
- Add the chicken breasts and sauce into the slow cooker.
- Cover with lid and cook on low heat for 7 hours.

- Allow the chicken to cool then shred the chicken with 2 forks.
- Place the chicken back into the slow cooker to absorb the sauce for an additional 30 minutes.
- Serve with pasta or quinoa.

21. Pulled Pork Pepper & Slaw Tacos

Yields: 12 servings

Ingredients:

4 lb. boneless pork shoulder

1 tsp. salt

1 tsp. black pepper

1 tbsp. canola oil

2 tbsp. chopped fresh parsley

1½ tsp. dried oregano

4 cloves garlic, chopped

2 cups chicken broth (fat free, low sodium)

½ cup apple cider vinegar

2 Anaheim peppers, seeded and sliced*

¼ tsp. crushed red pepper flakes

Slaw

12 (6-inch) corn tortillas

2 cups tricolor slaw mix

2 tbsp. fresh cilantro leaves

1½ tbsp. fresh lime juice

1 tbsp. olive oil

1 tsp. ground cumin

½ tsp. salt

Directions:

- Season pork with salt and pepper.
- Heat oil in a large skillet over high heat. Add pork; cook 5 minutes per side or until browned.
- Remove from heat and transfer to a 5- or 6-quart slow cooker. Add parsley, oregano, garlic, broth, vinegar, peppers and crushed red pepper flakes to slow cooker.
- Cover and cook on Low 6 to 8 hours or until pork is tender.
- Use half of the pork for Pork Tacos, and the other half can be frozen for the next time pork tacos are made or another pulled pork dish.

Prepare the Slaw

- Heat tortillas according to package instructions.
- Combine slaw mix, cilantro, lime juice, oil, cumin and salt in a medium bowl; toss to coat.
- Gently warm pork in a warm oven; shred with 2 forks. Arrange pork in tortillas; top with slaw.

Additional Reads and Recommendations

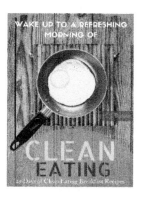

Wake Up to a Refreshing Morning of Clean Eating: 25 Days of Clean Eating Breakfast Recipes

Clean Eating: Amazingly Delicious Recipes To Jump Start Your Weight Loss, Increase Energy and Feel Great! (Clean Food Diet Book 1)

Clean Eating: Clean Eating Diet: The 7-Day Plan for Weight Loss & Delicious Recipes for Clean Eating Diet (Clean Eating, Weight Loss, Healthy Diet, Healthy ... Paleo Diet, Lose Weight Fast, Flat Belly)

CPSIA information can be obtained at www.ICGtesting.com
Printed in the USA
LVOW02s2343231015

459506LV00024BA/1130/P